Lean and Green Diet for Beginners

How to Eat Healthy and Weight Loss with 50 Low-Carb Delicious Recipes

By

Spoons of Happiness

policies, processes, or Instructions: contained within is the solitary and utter responsibility of the recipient reader. Under no circumstances will any legal responsibility or blame be held against the publisher for any reparation, damages, or monetary loss due to the information herein, either directly or indirectly.

Respective authors own all copyrights not held by the publisher.

The information herein is offered for informational purposes solely and is universal as such. The presentation of the information is without a contract or any type of guarantee assurance.

The trademarks that are used are without any consent and the publication of the trademark is without permission or backing by the trademark owner. All trademarks and brands within this book are for clarifying purposes only and are owned by the owners themselves, not affiliated with this document.

Table of Contents

Introduction

The Lean & Green diet is oriented towards the acquisition of a healthy and wholesome lifestyle, through the incorporation of pre-packaged products called "Fuelings". This diet seeks the transformation of lifelong eating habits by incorporating healthy practices, with the guidance of health coaching and the adoption of its dietary advice, as well as the Lean & Green products. The gradual replacement of "Fuelings" with a "Lean & Green" meal composed of balanced meat, vegetable, and a fat meal will keep you well-nourished and satiate hunger and cravings.

What is the Lean & Green diet all about?

Primarily, the Lean & Green diet is a weight loss and maintenance plan that combines a series of purchased, refined foods called "Fuelings" with low-fat, low-carbohydrate home-cooked meals.

One of its advantages is that you don't have to count carbohydrates or calories.

The idea is to take six or more mini-meals a day between fuelings and home-cooked meals. These meals include bars, shakes, cookies, cereals, soup, and mashed potatoes, all of which have soy protein or whey protein as the first ingredient.

The above foods are combined with 3 servings of non-starchy vegetables, 5-7 ounces of lean protein such as tuna, chicken, egg whites, turkey, or soy, and a maximum of 2 servings of balanced fat, such as olive oil, olives, or avocado.

Although it may not seem like it, the diet provides a reduced intake of carbohydrates. Because carbohydrates are the body's main source of energy, restricting them sends the body to use an alternative fuel source and starts burning fat. With the Lean & Green Diet, carbohydrate intake is reduced to 80-100 grams per day.

The Lean & Green diet brings many health benefits including weight loss by controlling portion sizes of meals and snacks, reducing the number of calories and carbohydrates. The menu reduces meal calories to 800-1000 calories per day and divides them into six regulated meal portions. Also, the Lean and Green diet helps improve blood pressure control by encouraging lower salt intake. With the Green and Lean diet, a lean and balanced body can be achieved with an easy and simple diet plan, avoiding hunger and cravings by consuming pre-packaged low-calorie foods and home-cooked meals.

Chapter 1: Snacks Recipes

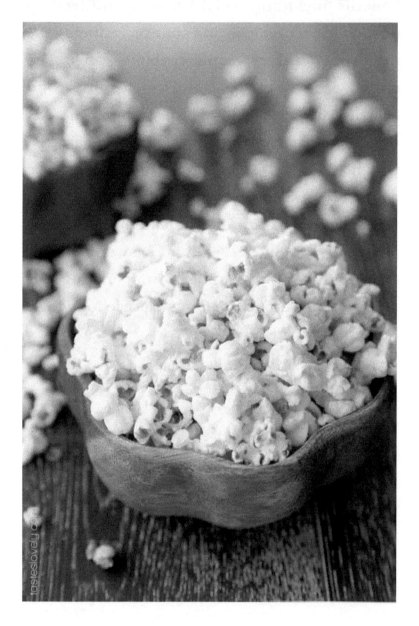

In this chapter, we are going to give you some delicious and mouthwatering recipes on Octavia Snacks recipes.

1. Kettle Corn

(Ready in 15 Minutes, Serve 4, Difficulty: Normal)

Nutrition per Serving:

Calories 209, Protein 2.4 g, Carbohydrates 24.8 g, Fat 11.9 g, Sodium 0.6mg.

Ingredients:

- ¼ cup of vegetable oil

- ¼ cup of white sugar

- ½ cup of unlopped popcorn kernels

Instructions:

1. Heat the vegetable oil in a big pot over a medium bowl. Stir in the popcorn and sugar until they have warmed up. To prevent the sugar from smoking, cover, shake the pot continuously before the popping has slowed to once, every 2-3 seconds.

2. Remove the pot from the heat and start shaking for a couple of minutes before the popping has stopped. Pour into a large bowl and allow to cool, frequently mixing to break up large clump

2. Coconut Cream Pops

(Ready in 10 Minutes, Serve 10, Difficulty: Normal)

Nutrition per Serving:

Calories 90, Protein 3 g, Carbohydrates 11 g, Fat 3.5 g, Sodium 44.5mg.

Ingredients:

- 1(12 fluid ounces) can of fat-free evaporated milk

- 1(13.5 ounces) can of light coconut milk

- ½ cup of confectioners' sugar

- 2 teaspoons of coconut extract

- Ground cinnamon, to taste

Instructions:

1. Whisk together the evaporated milk, coconut milk, confectioners' sugar, coconut extract, and ground cinnamon.

2. Pour into freezer pop molds, and freeze them until they are solid.

3. Potato Chips

(Ready in 10 Minutes, Serve 2, Difficulty: Normal)

Nutrition per Serving:

Calories 80, Protein 1.2 g, Carbohydrates 11.6 g, Fat 3.5 g, Sodium 294.5mg, Cholesterol mg.

Ingredients:

- 1 tablespoon of vegetable oil

- 1 potato, sliced paper-thin (Peeling is optional)

- ½ teaspoon of salt, or to taste

Instructions:

1. Through a plastic bag, pour vegetable oil (a produce bag works well). Add the slices of potatoes and shake to coat.

2. Lightly coat a large dinner plate with oil or cooking spray. Arrange the potato slices on the large plate in a single layer.

3. Cook for 3-5 minutes, or until gently browned in the microwave (if they are not browned, they will not become crisp). Depending on the microwave's power, time can vary.

4. Take the chips off the plate and toss them with salt (or other seasonings). Let it cool. Repeat the procedure with the remaining slices of potatoes. No need to continue to oil the plate.

4. Prosciutto e Malone (Italian Ham and Melon)

(Ready in 15 Minutes, Serve 6, Difficulty: Normal)

Nutrition per Serving:

Calories 99, Protein 3.9 g, Carbohydrates 11.3 g, Fat 4.8 g, Sodium 296.4mg, Cholesterol 12.5mg.

Ingredients:

- 1 cantaloupe, seeded and cut into 8 wedges

- 8 thin slices of prosciutto

Instructions:

1. Remove the tissue from the cantaloupe's rind.

2. Wrap a slice of ham for each piece of cantaloupe.

3. Serve it cold.

5. Baked Tortilla Chips

(Ready in 20 Minutes, Serve 6, Difficulty: Normal)

Nutrition per Serving:

Calories 147, Protein 3.3 g, Carbohydrates 26 g, Fat 4.1 g, Sodium 418mg.

Ingredients:

- 1(12 ounces) package of corn tortillas

- 1 tablespoon of vegetable oil

- 3 tablespoons of lime juice

- 1 teaspoon of ground cumin

- 1 teaspoon of chili powder

- 1 teaspoon of salt

Instructions:

1. Preheat the oven to 350 degrees Fahrenheit (176 degrees Celsius).

2. Break each tortilla into wedges of 8 chip sizes and place the wedges on a cookie sheet in a single layer.

3. Combine oil and lime juice in a mister. Mix well and spray until mildly moist with each tortilla wedge.

4. In a small dish, mix the chili powder, salt, and brush on the chips.

5. Bake for about 7 minutes. Rotate the pan and bake until the chips are crispy but not too brown, or for another 8 minutes.

6. Serve with garnishes, salsas, or guacamole.

Chapter 2: Breakfast Recipes

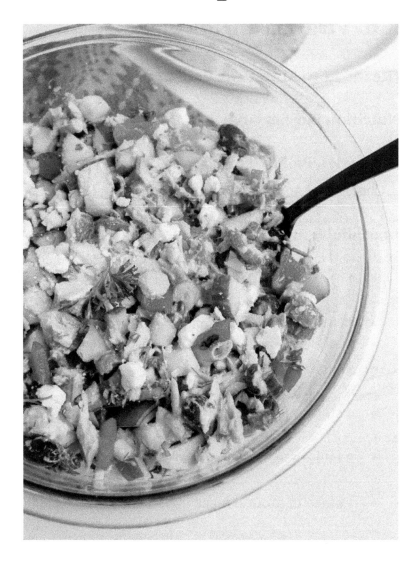

In this chapter, we are going to give you some delicious and mouthwatering recipes on Octavia Breakfast recipes.

6. Virginia's Tuna Salad

(Ready in 10 Minutes, Serve 2, Difficulty: Easy)

Nutrition per Serving:

Calories 121, Protein 9.9 g, Carbohydrates 3.9 g, Fat 9.8 g, Cholesterol 59.9mg, Sodium 167.5mg.

Ingredients:

- 1 egg

- 1 (5 ounces) can of tuna, drained and flaked

- 3 tablespoons of mayonnaise

- 2 stalks of celery, chopped

- 2 tablespoons of sweet pickle relish

- 1 pinch of ground black pepper

Instructions:

1. Put the egg in a saucepan and cover it with cold water.

2. Bring the water to a boil and remove it from the heat instantly.

3. Cover the egg and allow it rest for 10-12 minutes in hot water. Remove from the hot water and chill for about 5 minutes. Peel and chop into bite-sized bits.

4. Mix the tuna and mayonnaise in a medium dish. Mix the egg, celery, sauce, and black pepper.

7. Green Lentils and Rice Assyrian Style

(Ready in 40 Minutes, Serve 8, Difficulty: Normal)

Nutrition per Serving:

Calories 123, Protein 8.2 g, Carbohydrates 34.6 g, Fat 7.3 g, Cholesterol 0mg, Sodium 222.1mg.

Ingredients:

- 1 cup of dry green lentils

- 2 cups of water

- 4 tablespoons of divided olive oil

- 1 cup of basmati rice

- 1 large of onion, chopped

- ¾ teaspoon salt, or to taste

Instructions:

1. Place the lentils in a pan and cover them with water.

2. Bring to a rolling boil over high heat for 5 minutes, and then cover and remove it from the heat.

3. Meanwhile, in cold water, rinse the rice until the water is clean.

4. Over medium heat, heat 2 tablespoons of olive or vegetable oil in a skillet. For around 1 minute, whisk in the rice until the grains turn opaque and white, then add the lentils and water.

5. Carry the rice mixture to a simmer, then cover and reduce the heat for 5 minutes to medium-low. Stir once, then cover and further reduce the heat to a minimum.

6. Continue cooking, sealed, until the rice is soft, about 15 more minutes (do not remove the lid!).

7. Meanwhile, over medium heat, heat the remaining 2 tablespoons of oil in the skillet. Stir in the onion, and cook and stir for around 5 minutes until the onion is soft and translucent.

8. Reduce heat to medium-low and continue cooking and stirring, 15-20 minutes more until the onion is very soft and dark brown.

8. Stir in the caramelized onion when the rice is ready and season with salt.

8. Banana pancakes

(Ready in 40 Minutes, Serve 4, Difficulty: Normal)

Nutrition per Serving:

Calories 243, Protein 9 g, Carbohydrates 15 g, Fat 15 g, Saturates 2 g, Sugars 14 g, Fiber 4 g, Salt 0.3 g.

Ingredients:

- 1 large banana

- 2 medium eggs, beaten

- 1 pinch of baking powder (Gluten-free if coeliac)

- 1 splash of vanilla extract

- 1 teaspoon of oil

- 25 g of roughly chopped pecans

- 125 g of raspberries

Instructions:

1. Mash one large banana with a fork in a bowl until it resembles a dense paste.

2. Stir in 2 beaten eggs, a pinch of baking powder, and a splash of vanilla extract (Gluten-free if coeliac).

3. Over medium heat, heat a large non-stick frying pan or pancake pan and spray with ½ teaspoon of oil.

4. Spoon 2 pancakes into the pan with ½ the flour, cook each side for 1-2 minutes, then tip them onto a plate.

5. With another ½ teaspoon of oil and the remaining batter, repeat the process.

6. Use the 25 g of roughly chopped pecans and 125 g of raspberries to top the pancakes.

9. Cardamom & Peach Quinoa Porridge

(Ready in 40 Minutes, Serve 4, Difficulty: Normal)

Nutrition per Serving:

Calories 231, Protein 8 g, Carbohydrates 37 g, Fat 4 g, Saturates 1 g, Sugars 10 g, Fiber 6 g, Salt 0.2 g.

Ingredients:

- 75 g of quinoa

- 25 g of porridge oats

- 4 cardamom pods

- 250ml of unsweetened almond milk

- 2 ripe peaches, cut into slices

- 1 teaspoon of maple syrup

Instructions:

1. In a shallow saucepan, combine 250ml of water and 100ml of almond milk to the quinoa, oatmeal, and cardamom pods. Bring to a boil, then simmer gently, stirring regularly, for 15 minutes.

2. Pour in the remaining almond milk and cook until smooth for an additional 5 minutes.

3. Remove the pods of cardamom, spoon them into bowls or pots, then add the peaches and maple syrup to the end.

10. Kale, Tomato & Poached Egg on Toast

(Ready in 40 Minutes, Serve 3, Difficulty: Normal)

Nutrition per Serving:

Calories 251, Protein 15 g, Carbohydrates 18 g, Fat 12 g, Saturates 3 g, Sugars 2 g, Fiber 3 g, Salt 0.8 g.

Ingredients:

- 2 teaspoon of oil

- 100 g of ready-chopped kale

- 1 clove of garlic, crushed

- ½ teaspoon of chili flakes

- 2 large eggs

- 2 slices of multigrain bread

- 50 g of halved cherry tomatoes

- 15 g of crumbled feta

Instructions:

1. Adjust the heat so that a wide water pan is brought to a boil.

2. Heat the oil over medium-hot heat in a frying pan and add the kale, garlic, and chili flakes.

3. Cook for 4 minutes, stirring regularly until the kale starts to crisp and wilts to 1/2 its size. Set aside.

4. Water rises to a rolling boil, and the eggs are poached for 2 minutes. Toast the bread.

5. With a slotted spoon, remove the poached eggs and cover each slice of toast with half of the kale, the egg, the cherry tomatoes, and the feta.

Chapter 3: Lunch Recipes

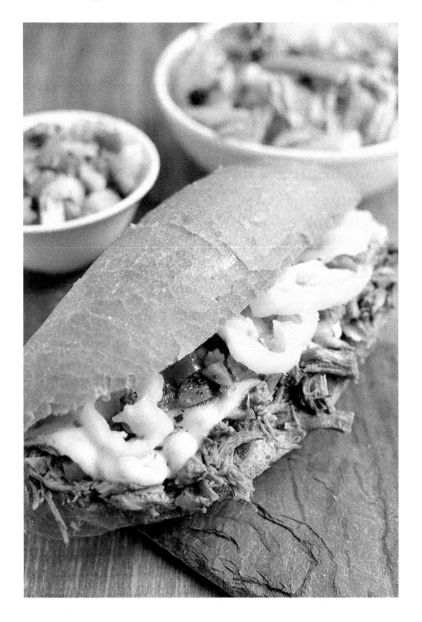

In this chapter, we are going to give you some delicious and mouthwatering recipes on Octavia Lunch recipes.

11. Slow Cooked Corned Beef for Sandwiches

(Ready in 4 Hours and 15 Minutes, Serve 1, and Difficulty: Normal)

Nutrition per Serving:

Calories 229, Protein 15 g, Carbohydrates 4.2 g, Fat 15.1 g, Cholesterol 77.9mg, Sodium 904.3mg.

Ingredients:

- 2(1360 g) of corned beef briskets with spice packets

- 2(12 fluid ounces) bottles of beer

- 2 bay leaves

- ¼ cup of peppercorns

- 1 bulb of clove garlic, separated and peeled

Instructions:

1. Place the briskets with the corned beef in a large pot. Sprinkle with 1 of the packets of spice and discard the other or save it for other uses. Pour in the beer and fill the saucepan with enough water to cover 1 inch of the briskets. Add the bay leaves, garlic, and peppercorns.

2. Reduce the heat to medium-low until the liquid comes to a boil, then simmer for 4-5 hours, checking hourly and adding more water if needed to keep the meat covered.

3. Remove the meat from the pot slowly, as it is going to be incredibly tender. Set it on a cutting board and allow it to rest for about 10 minutes before it firms up a little.

4. To serve, slice or shred, discard the cooking liquid, but it can be used for cooking cabbage and other vegetables if desired.

12. Basic Italian Bean Soup

(Ready in 25 Minutes, Serve 4, Difficulty: Normal)

Nutrition per Serving:

Calories 210, Protein 8.9 g, Carbohydrates 34.6 g, Fat 4.3 g, Cholesterol 0mg, Sodium 997.3mg.

Ingredients:

- Olive oil

- 1 large onion, diced

- 2 cloves of garlic, or more to taste

- 2 cups of tomato sauce

- 24 ounces of prepared cannellini beans

- 1 tablespoon of dried basil

- ½ teaspoon of oregano

- Salt and ground black pepper, to taste

Instructions:

1. Heat the olive oil over medium to high heat in a pot. In hot oil, cook and stir onion until tender, about 5 minutes, add garlic and proceed to cook until fragrant, about 1-2 more minutes.

2. Add the tomato sauce to the pot and stir. Add the peppers, basil, oregano, salt, and pepper to the cannellini.

3. Bring the mixture to a boil, reduce the heat to medium-low, and cook 5-7 more minutes until the beans are hot

13. Spicy Grilled Cheese Sandwich

(Ready in 5 Minutes, Serve 6, Difficulty: Easy)

Nutrition per Serving:

Calories 213, Protein 10.7 g, Carbohydrates 28.2 g, Fat 22.1 g, Cholesterol 57.2mg, Sodium 846.4mg.

Ingredients:

- 2 tablespoons of butter or margarine

- 4 slices of white bread

- 2 slices of American cheese

- 1 roman (plum) tomato, thinly sliced

- ¼ small onion, chopped

- 1 jalapeno pepper, chopped

Instructions:

1. Over low heat, heat a large skillet. Spread butter or margarine over 2 slices of bread on 1 side.

2. Place the buttered side of both pieces in the skillet. Place each one with a slice of cheese and top with the tomato, onion, and jalapeno strips.

3. Butter the remaining slices of bread on one side and put them on top of the buttered side. If the sandwiches are toasted at the bottom, flip and fry until the other side is brown.

14. Popular in Italian Recipes

(Ready in 1 Hour and 25 Minutes, Serve 4, And Difficulty: Hard)

Nutrition per Serving:

Calories 306, Protein 25.3 g, Carbohydrates 15.7 g, Fat 15.7 g, Cholesterol 78.7mg, Sodium 1398.8mg.

Ingredients:

- 680 g of boneless beef chuck, cut into 2-inch pieces

- Salt and ground black pepper, to taste

- 1 tablespoon of vegetable oil

- 6 cloves of garlic, sliced

- 2 tablespoons of white vinegar

- 1 tablespoon of dried oregano

- 1 ½ teaspoon of salt, or to taste

- 1 teaspoon of dried thyme

- 1 teaspoon of dried rosemary

- 1 teaspoon of freshly ground black pepper

- 1 bay leaf

- ¼ teaspoon of red pepper flakes, or to taste

- 3 cups of chicken broth, or as needed

- 4 ciabatta rolls, sliced in ½

- 1 cup of chopped giardiniera (pickled Italian vegetables)

- 2 teaspoons of chopped fresh flat-leaf parsley

Instructions:

1. Season the beef with a pinch of black pepper and salt. Heat the vegetable oil over high heat in a heavy pot. Cook and stir the beef until browned in hot oil, for 5-8 minutes.

2. Poon the beef with black pepper, bay leaf, and red pepper flakes. Pour enough chicken broth into the beef mixture to cover 1 inch of the meat and bring it to a simmer.

3. Cover the pot with a lid, reduce the heat to low, and simmer for 1-1 1/2 hour until the meat is fork-tender.

4. Transfer meat to a separate pot with a strainer or slotted spoon and pour about 1/4 cup of meat broth into the pot. To gently break the meat into smaller chunks, use a wooden spoon. Use a lid or aluminum foil to cover the pot and keep it warm.

5. Season with salt and pepper to taste. Skim the excess grease from the top of the broth remaining in the first pot. Use a lid or aluminum foil to cover the pot and keep the broth warm.

6. On a work surface, lay the halves of a rollout and spoon 2-3 tablespoons of meat broth over each 1/2. A generous portion of meat and a spoonful of pickled vegetables are on top of the roll's bottom ½. Place the top on the sandwich.

7. Repeat to create three more sandwiches with the remaining buns, broth, meat, and pickled vegetables.

8. Spoon the hot meat broth into ramekins and top 1/2 teaspoon of parsley with each ramekin. For dipping, serve sandwiches with hot broth.

15. Slow Cooker Italian Beef Sandwiches

(Ready in 8 Hours and 10 Minutes, Serve 1, and Difficulty: Hard)

Nutrition per Serving:

Calories 318, Protein 39.4 g, Carbohydrates 1.6 g, Fat 15.8 g, Cholesterol 100.4mg, Sodium 819.1mg.

Ingredients:

- 1(3721 g) rump roast

- 3 cups of water

- 2 tablespoons of dried basil

- 1 tablespoon of dried oregano

- 1 tablespoon of salt

- 1 tablespoon of garlic powder

- 1 tablespoon of parsley flakes

- 3 bay leaves

- 1 ½ teaspoons of red pepper flakes

- ⅓ teaspoon of ground black pepper, or to taste

Instructions:

1. In a slow cooker, combine the roast, basil, water, oregano, cinnamon, garlic powder, red pepper flakes, parsley flakes, bay leaves, and black pepper.

2. In a slow cooker, cook for 8-10 hours, set to low. Use 2 forks to remove bay leaves and shred beef.

16. Slow Cooker Spicy Black-Eyed Peas

Nutrition per Serving:

Calories 199, Protein 14.1 g, Carbohydrates 30.2 g, Fat 2.9 g, Cholesterol 9.6mg, Sodium 341.4mg.

(Ready in 6 Hours and 30 Minutes, Serve 10, and Difficulty: Hard)

Ingredients:

- 6 cups of water

- 1 cube of chicken bouillon

- 453 g of sorted, rinsed and, dried black-eyed peas

- 1 onion, diced

- 2 cloves of garlic, diced

- 1 red bell pepper, stemmed, seeded, and diced

- 1 jalapeno chile, seeded and minced

- 8 ounces of diced ham

- 4 slices of bacon, chopped

- ½ teaspoon of cayenne pepper

- 1 ½ teaspoon of cumin

- Salt, to taste

- 1 teaspoon of ground black pepper

Instructions:

1. Pour the water into a slow cooker to dissolve, add the bouillon cube, and stir.

2. Mix in the black-eyed peas, the onion, the jalapeno pepper, the garlic, the bell pepper, the ham, the cayenne pepper, the bacon, the salt, and the pepper, and mix well. Cover the slow cooker and simmer for 6-8 hours, until the beans are tender.

Chapter 4: Dinner Recipes

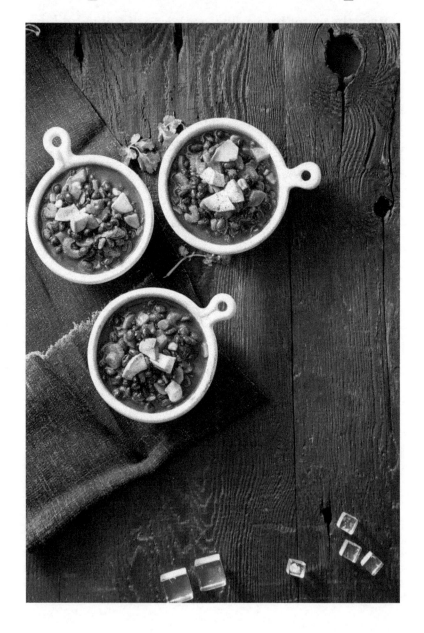

In this chapter, we are going to give you some delicious and mouthwatering recipes on Octavia Dinner recipes.

17. Smoky Vegan Black Bean Soup

(Ready in 4 Hours 50 Minutes, Serve 6, Difficulty: Hard)

Nutrition per Serving:

Calories 132, Protein 14 g, Carbohydrates 51 g, Fat 11 g, Saturated Fat 1 g, Fiber 19 g, Sodium 535mg.

Ingredients:

- 2 tablespoon of extra virgin olive oil

- 2 medium carrots, chopped

- 2 stalks of celery, sliced

- 1 medium onion, finely chopped

- ¼ cup of tomato paste

- 3 cloves of garlic, crushed with press

- 1 ½ teaspoon of ground cumin

- 1 teaspoon of smoked paprika

- 3 cups of lower-sodium vegetable or chicken broth

- 3 cans (15 oz. each) of lower-sodium black beans, undrained

- 1 cup of frozen corn

For Serving:

- Avocado chunks and cilantro leaves

Instructions:

1. In a 12-inch skillet, heat oil on medium-high. Add the carrots, onion, and celery. Cook for 6-8 minutes or until the browning begins, stirring occasionally.

2. Add the tomato paste, garlic, and paprika, all smoked. Cook, stirring, until the garlic is golden and the tomato paste is browned, or 1-2 minutes. Stir in half a cup of broth and scrape off any brown bits.

3. Skillet contents are transferred to the 6-8-quart slow-cooker bowl and beans, maize, and remaining broth. Cover and cook for 4 hours on high or 6 hours on low. Using avocado and cilantro to serve.

4. **Instant Pot Instructions**: As outlined in the step, select the cooking feature and cook vegetables. Add beans, maize, and broth, then. Select the slow cooking function and cook for 4 hours on high or 6 hours on low.

18. Salmon with Grilled Eggplant and Chickpea Croutons

(Ready in 1 Hour and 15 Minutes, Serve 4, Difficulty: Normal)

Nutrition per Serving:

Calories 330, Protein 37 g, Carbohydrates 29 g, Fat 19 g, Saturated Fat 3.5 g, Sodium 400 mg, Fiber 9 g.

Ingredients:

- 3 tablespoons plus 1 teaspoon of olive oil, divided

- 1 small onion, finely chopped

- 2 cloves of garlic, pressed, divided

- Kosher salt

- 1 cup of chickpea flour

- 1 tablespoon of lemon zest plus 2 teaspoons of lemon juice

- 2 medium eggplants (about 12 ounces each)

- 567 grams of skinless salmon fillet, cut into 4 pieces

- ¼ cup of plain full-fat yogurt

- 1 cup of mint leaves, torn

- 2 tablespoons of chopped chives

Instructions:

1. Line 4 1/2 with an 8 1/2-inch parchment loaf pan, leaving the overhang on 2 long sides. Heat 1 tablespoon of oil in a medium saucepan.

2. Add the onion, ½ the garlic, and ¼ teaspoon of salt, and cook until soft, occasionally stirring, for 5 minutes. Stir in 2 cups of water and bring it to a boil. Slowly stream in the chickpea flour when whisking and whisk vigorously, off the heat, until mostly lump-free.

3. Transfer the mixture with the lemon zest and puree to the food processor, gradually adding one tablespoon of oil until absolutely smooth. Transfer immediately to the prepared smooth top and pan. Cover and push with a heavy item with another sheet of parchment and another loaf pan. Refrigerate for 30 minutes to 1 hour until it is solid.

4. Meanwhile, heat a medium-high grill. Break the mixture of chickpeas into 1/2-inch cubes. In a small skillet, heat 1 teaspoon of oil and cook for 2-3 batches, occasionally turning, until browned, 3-5 minutes. Transfer to the paper towel to drain.

5. Slice the eggplants ½ inch thick lengthwise. Brush the remaining tablespoon of oil with the eggplant slices, season with a pinch of salt, and grill until tender and lightly charred, 3-4 minutes. Season salmon with ¼ teaspoon of salt and pepper each, add to grill along with eggplant, and grill 3-5 minutes per side until opaque throughout. Transferring to plates.

6. Whisk together the yogurt, lemon juice, remaining garlic, and a pinch of salt in a small bowl. Drizzle the eggplant with the yogurt sauce and sprinkle with the chickpea croutons, mint, and chives.

7. Serve with grilled salmon.

19. Mediterranean Chicken Bowls

(Ready in 20 Minutes, Serve 6, Difficulty: Normal)

Nutrition per Serving:

Calories 237, Protein 43 g, Carbohydrate 53 g, Fat 9.5 g, Saturated Fat 1.5 g, Sodium 425mg, Fiber 5 g.

Ingredients:

- 453 grams of boneless, skinless chicken breasts, cut into 1 ½-in pieces

- 1 tablespoon of olive oil

- 1 teaspoon of dried oregano

- 1 teaspoon of ground sumac

- Kosher salt and pepper

- 1 pint of grape or cherry tomatoes

- 1 medium onion, roughly chopped

- 1 cup of couscous

- 1 teaspoon of grated lemon zest plus

- 1 tablespoon of lemon juice

- ¼ cup of fresh dill, divided

For Serving:

- Crumbled feta

- Lemon wedges

Instructions:

1. Toss the chicken with the oil in a large bowl, then add the oregano, sumac, and ½ teaspoon of salt and pepper. Add the onion and tomatoes and toss to mix.

2. Arrange an even layer in the air fryer basket and fry at 400 degrees Fahrenheit (204 Celsius), shaking the basket occasionally, 15-20 minutes, until chicken is golden brown and cooked through.

3. In the meantime, toss couscous with lemon zest and prepare the directions per box. Fork and fold the fluff with lemon juice and 2 teaspoons of dill.

4. Serve over couscous chicken and vegetables, spooning over the top of any juices collected at the bottom of the air fryer. If desired, sprinkle with the remaining dill and feta and serve with lemon wedges.

20. Pan-Fried Chicken with Lemony Roasted Broccoli

(Ready in 35 Minutes, Serve 6, Difficulty: Easy)

Nutrition per Serving:

Calories 316, Protein 44 g, Carbohydrates 15 g, Fat 15.5 g, Saturated Fat 2.5 g, Sodium 375mg, Fiber 5 g.

Ingredients:

- 680 grams of broccoli, cut into florets

- 2 cloves of garlic, thinly sliced

- 3 tablespoon of olive oil

- Kosher salt and pepper

- 4 6-ounces of skinless-boneless chicken breast

- 1 cup of all-purpose flour

- 1 lemon, cut into ½-inch pieces

- 2 tablespoon of lemon juice

Instructions:

1. Heat the oven to 425 degrees Fahrenheit (218 degree Celsius). Toss the broccoli and garlic with 1 tablespoon of oil on the rimmed baking sheet. Roast for 10 minutes and add ¼ teaspoon of salt and pepper each.

2. Meanwhile, season with ¼ teaspoon of salt and pepper, chicken breasts to even thickness, then coat in flour. Heat 1 tablespoon of oil in a large skillet over medium-high heat and cook 3-5 minutes per side of chicken until golden brown. Nestle chicken in the center of broccoli and roast for about 6 minutes until chicken is cooked through and broccoli is golden brown and tender.

3. Return the skillet to medium heat, add the remaining tablespoons of oil, then the lemon bits, and cook for 3 minutes, stirring, until golden. Add lemon juice and 1/3 cup water and cook any browned pieces, stirring and scraping. Spoon and serve with broccoli over chicken.

4. Prepare and store the broccoli and lemons for up to 2 days before cooking.

21. Steak Salad with Charred Green Onions and Beets

(Ready in 35 Minutes, Serve 4, Difficulty: Easy)

Nutrition per Serving:

Calories 312, Protein 29 g, Carbohydrates 9 g, Fat 18 g, Sodium 735mg, Fiber 3 g.

Ingredients:

- 1(2" thick) of boneless top loin beefsteak (453 grams)

- 1 tablespoon of vegetable oil

- ½ bunch of green onions, halved

- ¾ teaspoon of flaky sea salt

- 1 ½ ounce of container mixed greens

- ½ small head radicchio, leaves separated and torn

- 4 cooked beets, quartered

- ¼ cup of red-wine vinegar

- 1 tablespoon of extra virgin olive oil

- 2 ounces of blue cheese, crumbled

Instructions:

1. Set up the sous vide unit in the 8-quart saucepot as the package directs. Add water and set the device's temperature to 130 degrees Celsius (266 degree F).

2. Place the steak in a reseal able plastic bag of a gallon size, seal tightly, push out excess air. Place your bag in hot water. Cook for 2 hours. Remove the bag from the water. Take the steak out of the bag and pat it dry.

3. Heat oil to medium-high until very hot in a 10-inch skillet. Add the green onions and cook for 2 minutes or until lightly charred. Add steak to skillet. Cook 2 minutes, turning frequently. Transfer to a cutting board, sprinkle with ½ teaspoon flaky sea salt, and thickly slice.

4. Toss the greens, radicchio, olive oil, beets, vinegar, and 1/4 teaspoon each of the flaky sea salt and pepper into a large cup. Transfer to a tray. Place the steak, onions, and blue cheese on top.

22. Tuna Poke Bowl Recipe

(Ready in 20 Minutes, Serve 6, Difficulty: Easy)

Nutrition per Serving:

Calories 200, Protein 29 g, Carbohydrate 7 g, Fat 5 g, Saturated Fat 1 g, Sodium 905 mg.

Ingredients:

- 1 tablespoon plus 1 teaspoon of low-sodium soy sauce

- 1 tablespoon plus 1 teaspoon of toasted sesame oil

- ¼ sweet onion, thinly sliced

- 3 scallions, thinly sliced

- Kosher salt

- 453 grams of fresh sushi-grade ahi tuna, cut into 1-inch cubes

- 1 Persian cucumber, thinly sliced

- 1 tablespoon of rice vinegar

- ¼ teaspoon of sugar

- 1 teaspoon of black sesame seeds, plus more for sprinkling

- 1 ripe avocado, quartered

For Serving:

- Cooked rice

Instructions:

1. Combine the soy sauce, onion, sesame oil, scallions, and a pinch of salt in a large bowl. Toss and refrigerate with tuna until ready for use.

2. Toss the cucumbers with sugar, vinegar, sesame seeds, and a pinch of salt in a small cup. Let the 5 minutes stand.

3. When needed, marinated cucumbers, serve tuna and avocado over rice. If needed, sprinkle with extra black sesame seeds.

Chapter 5: Soups Recipes

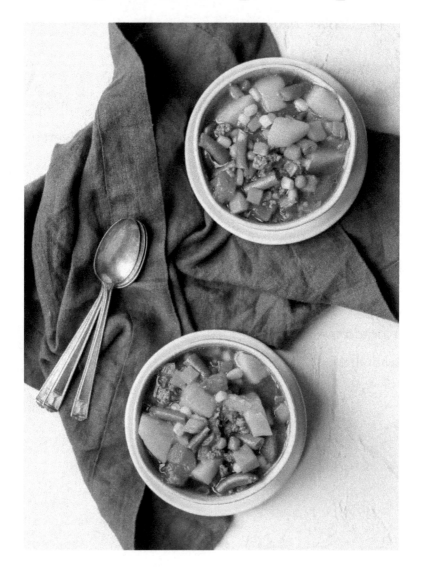

In this chapter, we are going to give you some delicious and mouthwatering recipes on Octavia Soups recipes.

23. Instant Pot® Hamburger Soup

(Ready in 1 Hour and 10 Minutes, Serve 8, Difficulty: Normal)

Nutrition per Serving:

Calories 112, Protein 18.7 g, Carbohydrates 17.8 g, Fat 11.2 g, Cholesterol 51.7mg, Sodium 950.4mg.

Ingredients:

- 680 g of ground beef

- 1 medium onion, finely chopped

- 3(14.5 ounces) cans of beef consommé

- 1(28 ounces) can of diced tomatoes

- 2 cups of water

- 1(10.75 ounces) can of condensed tomato soup

- 4 carrots, finely chopped

- 3 stalks of celery, finely chopped

- 4 tablespoons of pearl barley

- ½ teaspoon of dried thyme

- 1 bay leaf

Instructions:

1. Switch on a multi-functional pressure cooker and select the cook mode (such as Instant Pot®). Cook and stir until browned, 5-10 minutes, with the beef and onion. Pour the beef, onions, water, and tomato soup into the mixture. Add some celery, onions, barley, thyme, and bay leaf.

2. Cover the lid and lock it. Pick "Feature Soup," set the timer to 30 minutes. Allow pressure to build for 10-15 minutes.

3. The release pressure is about 10 minutes using the natural-release method as instructed by the manufacturer.

24. Cauliflower-Cheese Soup

(Ready in 45 Minutes, Serve 4, Difficulty: Normal)

Nutrition per Serving:

Calories 138, Protein 15.7 g, Carbohydrates 25.9 g, Fat 24.7 g, Cholesterol 74.9mg, Sodium 367.6mg.

Ingredients:

- ¾ cup of water

- 1 cup of chopped cauliflower

- 1 cup of cubed potatoes

- ½ cup of finely chopped celery

- ½ cup of diced carrots

- ¼ cup of chopped onion

- ¼ cup of butter

- ¼ cup of all-purpose flour

- 3 cups of milk

- Salt and pepper, to taste

- 4 ounces of shredded cheddar cheese

Instructions:

1. Combine the water, cauliflower, carrots, potatoes, celery, and onion in a large saucepan. It should be boiled for 5-10 minutes, or until tender. Only put aside.

2. Over medium pressure, melt the butter in a separate saucepan. Add the flour, then simmer for 2 minutes.

3. Remove from the heat, and stir in the milk gradually. Return to the heat and simmer until the mixture thickens. With the cooking liquid, stir in the vegetables and season with salt and pepper. Remove from the heat and whisk in the cheese until melted.

25. Chef John's Butternut Bisque

(Ready in 50 Minutes, Serve 6, Difficulty: Normal)

Nutrition per Serving:

Calories 213, Protein 3.2 g, Carbohydrates 27.1 g, Fat 13.7 g, Cholesterol 45.8mg, Sodium 1058.9mg.

Ingredients:

- 3 tablespoons of butter

- 1 large onion, diced

- 1 teaspoon of kosher salt, plus more to taste, divided

- 1(907 g) butternut squash

- 2 tablespoons of tomato paste

- 1 quart of chicken broth

- 1 pinch of cayenne pepper

- 2 tablespoons of maple syrup, or to taste

- ½ cup of heavy cream or crème fraiche

- Pomegranate seeds

For Garnish:

- Some heavy cream or crème fraiche

- Chopped fresh chives.

Instructions:

1. Over medium-low pressure, melt butter in a pot. Put in the onions and a huge pinch of salt. Cook and stir until the onions, around 10-15 minutes, have softened but not taken on any color.

2. Cut off the squash ends. Carefully cut the squash lengthwise in ½ and remove the seeds. Using a potato peeler, peel the squash. Slice into chunks.

3. Raise the heat to medium-high below the pot. In the tomato paste, stir, simmer, and stir until the mixture starts to caramelize and brown for about 2 minutes. Add the potato, 1 teaspoon of salt, chicken broth, and cayenne pepper. Bring to a boil, reduce heat to medium-low, and simmer, 15-25 minutes, until the squash is very tender. Reduce heat to low levels. Blend until very creamy with an immersion blender. Add the cream and maple syrup and if needed, add more salt.

4. Ladle into bowls for serving. garnish with a cream swirl and a scattering of pomegranate seeds and chives.

26. Sweet Potato, Carrot, Apple, and Red Lentil Soup

(Ready in 1 Hour and 10 Minutes, Serve 6, Difficulty: Normal)

Nutrition per Serving:

Calories 232, Protein 9 g, Carbohydrates 52.9 g, Fat 9 g, Cholesterol 21.6mg, Sodium 876.3mg.

Ingredients:

- ¼ cup of butter

- 2 large sweet potatoes, peeled and chopped

- 3 large carrots, peeled and chopped

- 1 apple, peeled, cored, and chopped

- 1 onion, chopped

- ½ cup of red lentils

- ½ teaspoon of minced fresh ginger

- ½ teaspoon of ground black pepper

- 1 teaspoon of salt

- ½ teaspoon of ground cumin

- ½ teaspoon of chili powder

- ½ teaspoon of paprika

- 4 cups of vegetable broth

- Plain yogurt

Instructions:

1. Melt the butter over medium-high heat in a big heavy-bottomed pot. In the pot, combine the chopped sweet potatoes, carrots, apple, and onion. Stir and cook the apples and vegetables for about 10 minutes before the onions are translucent.

2. In a pot with the apple and vegetable mixture, stir the lentils, ginger, ground black pepper, cinnamon, chili powder, paprika, and vegetable broth. Bring the soup to a boil over high heat, then reduce the heat to medium-low, cover and simmer for about 30 minutes until the lentils and vegetables are soft.

3. Pour the soup into a blender, working in batches, filling the pitcher no more than halfway full. With a folded kitchen towel, keep the blender's lid down and start the blender carefully, using a few short pulses to transfer the soup before leaving it to puree. Purée until smooth and pour into a clean pot in batches. Alternately, right in the cooking pot, you should use a stick blender to puree the broth.

4. Place the pureed soup back in the cooking pot. Bring back over medium-high heat, around 10 minutes, to a simmer. To thin the soup to your desired consistency, add water as needed. For garnish, serve with yogurt.

5. Instead of yogurt as a garnish, this soup is also well served with crumbled feta cheese.

27. California Italian Wedding Soup

(Ready in 25 Minutes, Serve 6, Difficulty: Easy)

Nutrition per Serving:

Calories 159, Protein 11.5 g, Carbohydrates 15.4 g, Fat 5.6 g, Cholesterol 55.3mg, Sodium 98.6mg.

Ingredients:

- 226 g of extra-lean ground beef

- 1 egg, lightly beaten

- 2 tablespoons of Italian-seasoned breadcrumbs

- 1 tablespoon of grated parmesan cheese

- 2 tablespoons of shredded fresh basil leaves

- 1 tablespoon of chopped Italian flat-leaf parsley (Optional)

- 2 green onions, sliced (Optional)

- 5 ¾ cups of chicken broth

- 2 cups of finely sliced escarole (spinach may be substituted)

- 1 lemon, zested

- ½ cup of orzo (rice-shaped pasta), uncooked

For Topping:

- Grated parmesan cheese

Instructions:

1. The meat, egg, parsley, bread crumbs, cheese, basil, and green onions are mixed to form 3/4-inch balls.

2. Over high heat, pour the broth into a large saucepan. Drop into meatballs while boiling. Stir in escarole, orzo, and lemon zest. Return to a boil and reduce to medium heat. Cook for 10 minutes on a slow boil or until the orzo is tender, stirring frequently. Serve with cheese.

28. Vegetarian Kale Soup

(Ready in 55 Minutes, Serve 8, Difficulty: Normal)

Nutrition per Serving:

Calories 277, Protein 9.6 g, Carbohydrates 50.9 g, Fat 4.5 g, Cholesterol 0mg, Sodium 372.2mg.

Ingredients:

- 2 tablespoons of olive oil

- 1 yellow onion, chopped

- 2 tablespoons of chopped garlic

- 1 bunch of kale, stems removed and leaves chopped

- 8 cups of water

- 6 cubes of vegetable bouillon (such as Knorr®)

- 1(15 ounces) can of diced tomatoes

- 6 white potatoes, peeled and cubed

- 2(15 ounces) cans of cannellini beans (drained if desired)

- 1 tablespoon of Italian seasoning

- 2 tablespoons of dried parsley

- Salt and pepper, to taste

Instructions:

1. In a large soup pot, heat the olive oil and cook the onion and garlic until soft. Stir in the kale and cook for about 2 minutes, until wilted. Stir in the water, stir up the water

2. Tomatoes, potatoes, beans, vegetable bouillon, Italian seasoning, and parsley. Simmer the soup for 25 minutes on medium heat or until the potatoes are fully cooked. To taste, season with salt and pepper.

Chapter 6: Vegan Recipes

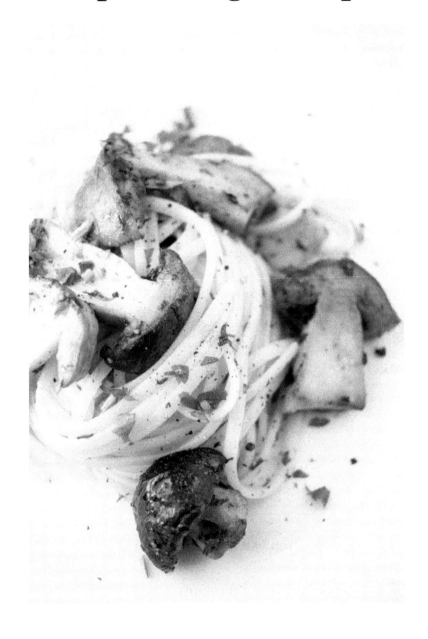

In this chapter we are going to give you some delicious and mouthwatering recipes on Octavia Vegan recipes.

29. Porcini Mushroom Pasta

(Ready in 55 Minutes, Serve 6, Difficulty: Normal)

Nutrition per Serving:

Calories 335, Protein 13.8 g, Carbohydrates 560.1 g, Fat 4.3 g, Cholesterol 0mg, Sodium 18.6mg.

Ingredients:

- 1 tablespoon of olive oil

- 2 cloves of garlic, minced

- ½ red onion, minced

- ½ cup of red bell pepper, julienned

- ½ cup of julienned carrots

- ½ cup of dry red wine

- 1 cup of rehydrated porcini mushrooms

- 1 ½ cup of crushed tomatoes

- 2 teaspoons of chopped fresh basil

- 1 teaspoon of dried rosemary, crushed

- Salt and pepper, to taste

- 6 cups of tagliatelle

Instructions:

1. Over medium heat, heat the oil in a large skillet. Add the onions and garlic and cook for 4 minutes, then add the red bell pepper and carrots and cook for another 4 minutes. Add the red wine, increase the heat, cook for 1 minute, reduce the heat to medium-low, add the mushrooms, and cook for 3 minutes.

2. Add the tomatoes, basil, and rosemary, season to taste with salt and pepper.

3. Simmer for 10 minutes, then serve over fried noodles with sauce.

30. Black-Eyed Peas and Tortillas

(Ready in 25 Minutes, Serve 4, Difficulty: Normal)

Nutrition per Serving:

Calories 287, Protein 15.1 g, Carbohydrates 76.8 g, Fat 13.2 g, Cholesterol 0mg, Sodium 1248.8mg.

Ingredients:

- 1 tablespoon olive oil

- ¼ cup finely chopped onion

- 1(15.5 ounces) can black-eyed peas, drained

- ½ cup vegetable stock

- 1 fresh jalapeno pepper, chopped

- 1 clove of garlic, minced

- 1 tablespoon of fresh lime juice

- Salt and pepper, to taste

- 4(12 inches) flour tortillas

Instructions:

1. Heat the olive oil over medium heat in a medium skillet and cook the onion until it is tender.

2. Combine the black-eyed peas, vegetable reserve, jalapeno, lime juice, and garlic cloves. Season to taste with salt and pepper, and continue cooking until hot.

3. Wrap the mixture in the tortillas to serve.

31. Spicy Couscous with Dates

(Ready in 30 Minutes, Serve 2, Difficulty: Easy)

Nutrition per Serving:

Calories 129, Protein 18 g, Carbohydrates 111.9 g, Fat 10.6 g, Cholesterol 0mg, Sodium 314.5mg.

Ingredients:

- 2 whole star anise pods

- Salt, to taste

- 3 cloves of garlic, peeled and chopped

- ½ red bell pepper, chopped

- 2 dried hot red peppers, diced

- ½ teaspoon of ground black pepper

- 4 large fresh mushrooms, chopped

- 1 tablespoon of lemon juice

- ¼ cup of chopped dates

- 1 teaspoon of ground cinnamon

- 1 cup of uncooked couscous

- 1 ½ cups of vegetable stock

Instructions:

1. Heat the oil over low heat in a medium saucepan, and sauté the onion until it is tender. Using the anise pods and salt to season. Blend the garlic, red bell pepper, spicy dried red peppers, and black pepper. Continue to cook and stir until you have tender vegetables.

2. Stir in the vegetable mixture with the mushrooms and lemon juice. Add in the dates and cinnamon, and cook for around 10 minutes over low heat.

3. In a medium saucepan, position the couscous and cover with vegetable supply. Bring it to a boil. Reduce heat to low levels. Cover and boil until the moisture has been drained, 3-5 minutes.

4. With a fork, mix in the vegetables and eat. Fluff couscous.

32. Oven Roasted Red Potatoes and Asparagus

(Ready in 1 Hour, Serve 6, Difficulty: Normal)

Nutrition per Serving:

Calories 149, Protein 4.2 g, Carbohydrates 23.5 g, Fat 4.9 g, Cholesterol 0mg, Sodium 650.5mg.

Ingredients:

- 680 g of red potatoes, cut into chunks

- 2 tablespoons of extra virgin olive oil

- 8 cloves of garlic, thinly sliced

- 4 teaspoons of dried rosemary

- 4 teaspoons of dried thyme

- 2 teaspoons of kosher salt

- 1 bunch of fresh asparagus, trimmed and cut into 1-inch pieces

- Ground black pepper to taste

Instructions:

1. Preheat oven to 425 degrees Fahrenheit (218 degrees Celsius).

2. In a large baking dish, toss the red potatoes with ½ the olive oil, garlic, rosemary, thyme, and ½ the kosher salt. Cover with aluminum foil.

3. Bake 20 minutes in the preheated oven. Mix in the asparagus, remaining olive oil, and remaining salt. Cover, and continue cooking 15 minutes, or until the potatoes are tender. Increase oven temperature to 450 degrees Fahrenheit (232 degrees Celsius).

4. Remove foil, and continue cooking 5-10 minutes, until potatoes are lightly browned. Season with pepper to serve.

33. Vegan Holiday Roast with Mashed Vegetables

(Ready in 10 Minutes, Serve 4-6, Difficulty: Easy)

Nutrition per Serving:

Calories 246, Protein 19 g, Carbohydrates 22 g, Fat 9 g, Fiber 3g.

Ingredients:

- 1, 1 lb. (thawed) vegan stuffed roast

- 2 cups diced potato

- 2 cups diced carrots

- 1 cup diced yellow onion

- ¾-1 cup of veggie broth

- 4 minced garlic cloves

- 1 tablespoon almond milk

- 1 teaspoon olive oil

- Salt and pepper to taste

Instructions:

1. In your pressure cooker, heat the oil.

2. Cook the garlic and onion for 1 minute when it is hot.

3. Add the vegetables, salt, and potatoes and combine.

4. On top of the vegetables, put the roast on top and spill over the broth.

5. Cover the lid and seal it

6. Select 'manual' and cook for 8 minutes at low pressure or around 6 minutes at high pressure.

7. Hit 'cancel' and quick-release when the time is up.

8. Let the roast out.

9. For the vegetables, add almond milk and pepper and mash to your perfect consistency.

10. Serve.

34. Spinach, Red Lentil, and Bean Curry

(Ready in 35 Minutes, Serve 4, Difficulty: Easy)

Nutrition per Serving:

Calories 328, Protein 18 g, Carbohydrates 51.9 g, Fat 8.3 g, Cholesterol 1.7mg, Sodium 633mg.

Ingredients:

- 1 cup of red lentils

- ¼ cup of tomato puree

- ½ (8 ounces) container of plain yogurt

- 1 teaspoon of garam masala

- ½ teaspoon of ground dried turmeric

- ½ teaspoon of ground cumin

- ½ teaspoon of Ancho chile powder

- 2 tablespoons of vegetable oil

- 1 onion, chopped

- 2 cloves of garlic, chopped

- 1(1 inch) piece fresh ginger root, grated

- 4 cups of loosely packed fresh spinach, coarsely chopped

- 2 tomatoes, chopped

- 4 sprigs of fresh cilantro, chopped

- 1(15.5 ounces) can of mixed beans, rinsed and drained.

Instructions:

1. Rinse the lentils and put enough water in a saucepan to cover them. Bring it to a boil. Lower the heat, cover the kettle and boil for 20 minutes over low heat, drain.

2. Stir the tomato puree and yogurt together in a dish. Season with garam masala, turmeric, chili powder, and cumin. Remove before creamy.

3. Heat oil over low heat in a pan. Add the onion, garlic, and ginger, then simmer until the onion starts to brown. Stir in the spinach, then simmer until wilted and dark green. Stir in the yogurt mixture gradually. Then the tomatoes and cilantro are combined.

4. Stir in the mixture of lentils and mixed beans once well balanced. Heat through, 5 minutes, approximately.

Chapter 7: Meat Dishes

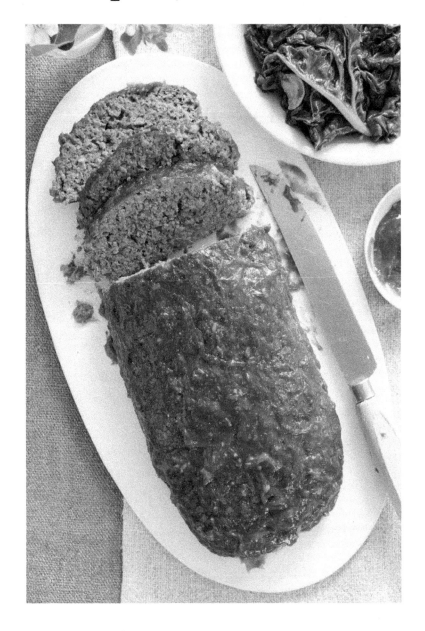

In this chapter, we are going to give you some delicious and mouthwatering recipes on Lean & Green Meat Dishes recipes.

35. Glazed Meatloaf II

(Ready in 1 Hour and 20 Minutes, Serve 8, Difficulty: Hard)

Nutrition per Serving:

Calories 318, Protein 22.4 g, Carbohydrates 18.9 g, Fat 16.8 g, Cholesterol 89.7mg, Sodium 398.2mg

Ingredients:

- ½ cup of ketchup

- 1 cup of brown sugar

- 1 tablespoon of lemon juice

- 1 teaspoon of dry mustard

- 907 g of lean ground beef

- 3 slices of bread, shredded

- ¼ cup of diced onion

- 1 egg, beaten

- 1 cube of beef bouillon, crumbled

- 3 tablespoons of lemon juice

Instructions:

1. Preheat the oven to 350 degrees Fahrenheit (176 degrees Celsius).

2. Combine the ketchup, brown sugar, 1 tablespoon of lemon juice, and the dried mustard in a small bowl until smooth.

3. Combine ground beef, egg, bouillon, shredded bread, onion, 3 tablespoons lemon juice, and 1/3 cup ketchup mixture in a large bowl until well blended. In a 9x5-inch loaf pan, form into a loaf and place.

4. Bake for one hour. Pour the fat away. Pour a mixture of reserved ketchup over the loaf. Bake for an extra 10 minutes.

36. Bacon-Wrapped Buffalo Meatloaf

(Ready in 2 Hours. Serve 6, Difficulty: Easy)

Nutrition per Serving:

Calories 348, Protein 35.8 g, Carbohydrates 19.3 g, Fat 13.6 g, Cholesterol 134.5mg, Sodium 1239.3mg.

Ingredients:

- 2 tablespoons of butter

- 2 slices of bacon, chopped

- ½ yellow onion, chopped

- 1 carrot, cubed

- 1 red bell pepper, chopped

- 1 fresh poblano pepper, chopped (Optional)

- 4 button mushrooms, chopped

- 3 cloves of garlic

- ¼ teaspoon of dried rosemary

- 2 cups of fresh bread crumbs

- ¼ cup of milk

- 1 large egg

- 2 teaspoons of kosher salt, or to taste

- 1 teaspoon of Worcestershire sauce

- 1 teaspoon of freshly ground black pepper

- 1 pinch of cayenne pepper

- 907 g of ground buffalo

- 7 slices of thick-cut bacon, or more as needed

For Glaze:

- 2 tablespoons of rice vinegar (optional)

- 2 tablespoons of brown sugar (optional)

- 1 tablespoon of Dijon mustard (optional)

Instructions:

1. Preheat the oven to 350 degrees Fahrenheit (176 degrees Celsius). Grease a 9x13-inch baking dish lightly.

2. Melt butter over medium heat in a large skillet. Cook and stir the chopped bacon in the hot butter for 5-10 minutes, until almost crisp.

3. In a food processor, slice the onion, carrot, poblano pepper, celery, red bell pepper, mushrooms, and garlic until finely chopped.

4. In the skillet, add the vegetable blend and rosemary to the bacon, cook and stir until the vegetables are softened and sweetened, about 5 minutes.

5. In a bowl, combine the vegetable mixture, bread crumbs, and milk. Let the room temperature cool. Stir in the vegetable mixture, egg, salt, Worcestershire sauce, black pepper, and cayenne pepper. Add the buffalo meat to the vegetable mixture and blend until well blended with your hands.

6. Turn the meat mixture into a prepared baking dish and form a 9x5x3-inch meatloaf. Lay bacon strips crosswise over the meatloaf's top, tucking bacon beneath the loaf at the ends.

7. In a bowl, whisk together the rice vinegar, brown sugar, and mustard until the glaze is soft.

8. Bake the meatloaf for 30 minutes in a preheated oven. Brush the glaze over the loaf and continue baking until the center is no longer pink, about 30 more minutes. A center-inserted instant-read thermometer should read at least 155 degrees Fahrenheit (68 degrees Celsius), before slicing, cool for 10 minutes.

37. Mini Meatloaves

(Ready in 1 Hour, Serve 8, Difficulty: Normal)

Nutrition per Serving:

Calories 325, Protein 15.1 g, Carbohydrates 16.6 g, Fat 14.4 g, Cholesterol 73.9mg, Sodium 656mg.

Ingredients:

- 1 egg

- ¾ cup of milk

- 1 cup of shredded cheddar cheese

- ½ cup of quick-cooking oats

- 1 teaspoon of salt

- 453 g of ground beef

- ⅔ cup of ketchup

- ¼ cup of packed brown sugar

- 1 ½ teaspoon of prepared mustard

Instructions:

1. Preheat the oven to 350 degrees Fahrenheit (176 degrees Celsius).

2. Combine the egg, milk, cheese, oatmeal, and salt in a large bowl. Add the ground beef, mix well, and make eight miniature meatloaves to form this mixture.

3. Place these in a 9x13 inch baking dish, which is lightly greased.

4. Combine the ketchup, brown sugar, and mustard in another small bowl. Stir and spread thoroughly over each meatloaf.

5. Bake, uncovered, for 45 minutes at 350 degrees Fahrenheit (176 degrees Celsius).

38. Instant Pot® Meatloaf

(Ready in 1 Hour and 25 Minutes, Serve 8, Difficulty: Hard)

Ingredients:

- 907 g of ground beef

- 1 cup of dry bread crumbs

- ½ cup of diced onion

- ½ apple, peeled, cored, and diced

- 2 teaspoons of garlic powder

- ½ teaspoon of salt

- ½ teaspoon of ground black pepper

For Topping:

- ⅓ cup of ketchup

- 2 tablespoons of prepared yellow mustard

- 2 tablespoons of brown sugar

Instructions:

1. In a large bowl, add the meat, bread crumbs, onion, apple, garlic powder, salt, and pepper until finely combined.

2. Shape a loaf with the beef mixture and put it on a large piece of aluminum foil. Fold the foil up and around the meatloaf's edges, producing a makeshift loaf pan.

3. In a multi-functional pressure cooker, pour 1/2 cup water (such as Instant Pot®) and place the steam rack inside with the handles up.

4. On the top of the rack, put the meatloaf. Seal the vent, close the lid, and lock it. According to the manufacturer's instructions, choose high pressure, and set the timer for 25 minutes. Allow pressure to build for 10 to 15 minutes.

5. Set a rack for the oven about 6 inches from the heat source and preheat the oven's broiler.

6. Use the quick-release method according to the manufacturer's instructions to carefully release cooker pressure for about 5 minutes. Unlock the lid and then remove it. Transfer the meatloaf to a baking sheet, still on the rack. Broil the meatloaf in the oven for about 5 minutes, until browned.

7. In a small bowl, combine your ketchup, mustard, and brown sugar. Brush over the meatloaf and broil again for 1-2 minutes, until caramelized.

39. Lighter Meatloaf

(Ready in 1 Hour and 35 Minutes, Serve 8, Difficulty: Normal)

Nutrition per Serving:

Calories 229, Protein 21.5 g, Carbohydrates 18.5 g, Fat 14.6 g, Cholesterol 71mg, Sodium 466.3mg.

Ingredients:

- Cooking spray

- 453 g of ground sirloin

- 453 g of ground turkey

- 1 cup of quick-cooking oats

- 1 small onion, chopped

- 2 large eggs

- 2 large white eggs

- 7 tablespoons of chili sauce, divided

- 1 tablespoon of dried basil

- 1 teaspoon of minced garlic from a jar

- ½ teaspoon of salt

- ½ teaspoon of coarsely ground black pepper

Instructions:

1. Preheat the oven to 375 degrees Fahrenheit (190 degrees Celsius). Using cooking spray to prepare a glass or stoneware 13x9-inch baking bowl.

2. In a bowl, mix the sirloin, turkey, egg whites, oats, onion, eggs, three tablespoons of chili sauce, basil,

garlic, salt, and pepper, turn into a 9x5-inch loaf, and place in the baking dish.

3. Bake for 50 minutes in the preheated oven. Spoon the leftover chili sauce over the top of the meatloaf and continue to bake for about 20 more minutes until the middle is no longer pink.

4. A center-inserted instant-read thermometer can read at least 160 degrees Fahrenheit (70 degrees Celsius). Before slicing, allow the meatloaf to rest for 10 minutes.

40. Italian Style Turkey Meatloaf

(Ready in 1 Hour and 5 Minutes, Serve 6, Difficulty: Hard)

Nutrition per Serving:

Calories 216, Protein 17.8 g, Carbohydrates 8.1 g, Fat 7 g, Cholesterol 86.8mg, Sodium 651mg.

Ingredients:

- Cooking spray

- 453 g of ground turkey

- 1 egg

- ¼ cup of Italian seasoned bread crumbs

- 1 teaspoon of Italian seasoning

- ½ clove of garlic, minced

- ½ teaspoon of ground black pepper, or to taste

- ¼ teaspoon of salt, or to taste

- 2 cups of tomato sauce, divided

Instructions:

1. Preheat oven to 400 degrees Fahrenheit (204 degrees Celsius). Prepare a baking dish with spray for cooking.

2. In a big cup, blend turkey, egg, bread crumbs, Italian seasoning, garlic, black pepper, salt, form a loaf, and place in a prepared baking dish.

3. Bake for 40 minutes in a preheated oven. Spoon over the loaf with around ½ the tomato sauce and proceed.

4. Bake for 10-15 more minutes, until the meatloaf is no longer pink in the middle. A center-inserted instant-read thermometer can read at least 160 degrees Fahrenheit (70 degrees Celsius). Set aside the meatloaf for 5-10 minutes before serving.

5. Serve with the cut meatloaf as the meatloaf sits, and cook the remaining tomato sauce over medium-low heat in a small saucepan.

Chapter 8: Salad Recipes

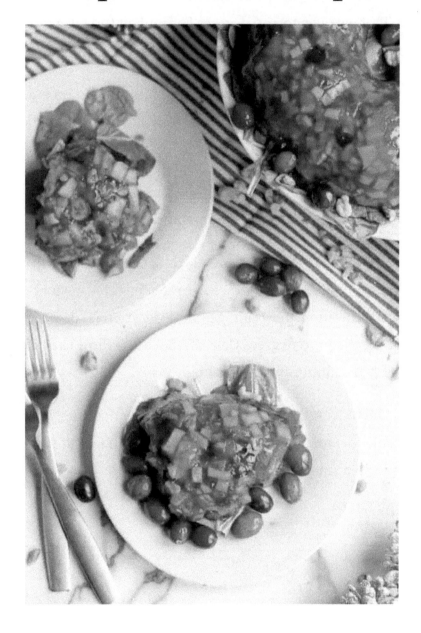

In this chapter we are going to give you some delicious and mouthwatering recipes on Lean & Green Salad recipes.

41. Cranberry Salad

(Ready in 15 Minutes, Serve 10, Difficulty: Easy)

Nutrition per Serving:

Calories 157, Protein 1.4 g, Carbohydrates 25.8 g, Fat 6.1 g, Cholesterol 0.6mg, Sodium 17.1mg.

Ingredients:

- 1(12 ounces) package of fresh cranberries, finely chopped

- ½ cup of white sugar

- 2 cups of chopped apples

- 1 cup of miniature marshmallows

- ½ cup of chopped pecans

- ½ cup of vanilla yogurt

- 1 cup of frozen whipped topping (such as Cool Whip®), thawed

Instructions:

1. In a large, non-reactive bowl, combine the chopped cranberries and sugar. Toss well.

2. For 3 hours cover and refrigerate.

42. Cranberry Salad II

(Ready in 20 Minutes, Serve 7, Difficulty: Easy)

Nutrition per Serving:

Calories 315, Protein 4.3 g, Carbohydrates 54.5 g, Fat 11 g, Cholesterol 0mg, Sodium 60.7mg.

Ingredients:

- 2 cups of cranberries

- 1 large orange

- 1 cup of white sugar

- 1 cup of finely chopped walnuts

- 1 cup of chopped celery

- 1 cup of crushed pineapple, drained

- 1(3 ounces) package of raspberry flavored Jell-O® mix

- 2 cups of hot water

Instructions:

1. Combine the gelatin (do not make it stand) with hot water. Mix cranberries with orange (including rind) and sugar. Stir in the almonds, pineapple, and celery.

2. Mix and chill with prepared gelatin.

43. Mom G's Cranberry Jell-O® Salad

(Ready in 4 Hours and 35 Minutes, Serve 8, and Difficulty: Normal)

Nutrition per Serving:

Calories 260, Protein 3.4 g, Carbohydrates 54.3 g, Fat 4.9 g, Cholesterol 0mg, Sodium 127.9mg.

Ingredients:

- 2(3 ounces) packages of lemon-flavored gelatin mix (such as Jell-O®)

- 1½ cup of boiling water

- 2 cups of cold water

- 1(12 ounces) package of fresh cranberries

- 1 cup of white sugar

- 1 cup of crushed pineapple, drained

- ¾ cup of chopped celery

- ½ cup of chopped walnuts

Instructions:

1. In a bowl of boiling water, dissolve the lemon gelatin and stir in cold water. Chill in the refrigerator for 30-40 minutes, before slightly thickened.

2. In a food processor, chop cranberries and blend sugar into cranberries, pulsating once or twice to combine. Let the cranberry mixture rest for a few minutes to remove the sugar.

3. Stir the mixture of cranberries, pineapple, celery, and walnuts into the jelly. Pour into a mold of gelatin or a serving bowl. Refrigerate for about 4 hours before fully set.

44. Deviled Egg Salad

(Ready in 10 Minutes, Serve 6, Difficulty: Easy)

Nutrition per Serving:

Calories 146, Protein 6.5 g, Carbohydrates 1.3 g, Fat 12.6 g, Cholesterol 215.5mg 7, Sodium 216.6mg.

Ingredients:

- ¼ cup of mayonnaise

- ¼ cup of finely chopped green onion

- ½ teaspoon of prepared yellow mustard

- ¼ teaspoon of salt

- ¼ teaspoon of garlic powder

- ¼ teaspoon of paprika

- ⅛ teaspoon of ground black pepper

- 6 hard-boiled eggs, peeled and chopped

Instructions:

1. In a bowl, stir together the mayonnaise, green onion, mustard, cinnamon, garlic powder, paprika, and black pepper until smooth.

2. Add the eggs, then carefully pour in the mayonnaise mixture to coat them.

45. Winter Fruit Salad with Lemon Poppy seed Dressing

(Ready in 35 Minutes, Serve 12, Difficulty: Normal)

Nutrition per Serving:

Calories 277, Protein 4.9 g, Carbohydrates 21 g, Fat 20.6 g, Cholesterol 8.7mg, Sodium 201.3mg.

Ingredients:

- ½ cup of white sugar

- ½ cup of lemon juice

- 2 teaspoons of diced onion

- 1 teaspoon of Dijon-style prepared mustard

- ½ teaspoon of salt

- 1 cup of vegetable oil

- 1 tablespoon of poppy seeds

- 1 head of romaine lettuce, torn into bite-size pieces

- 4 ounces of shredded Swiss cheese

- 1 cup of cashews

- ¼ cup of dried cranberries

- 1 apple, peeled, cored, and diced

- 1 pear, peeled, cored, and sliced

Instructions:

1. Put the sugar, mustard, lemon juice, onion, and salt together in a blender or food processor. Blend properly. Add oil in a slow process with the machine still running.

2. Steady flow until the mixture is dense and smooth. Add the poppy seeds and blend them for just a few more seconds.

3. Toss together the romaine lettuce, sliced Swiss cheese, dried cranberries, cashews, apple, and pear in a large serving dish. Just before eating, pour the dressing over the salad and toss to coat.

46. Autumn Waldorf salad

(Ready in 40 Minutes, Serve 2, Difficulty: Normal)

Nutrition per Serving:

Calories 312, Protein 3.2 g, Carbohydrates 70.3 g, Fat 5.5 g, Cholesterol 0mg, Sodium 54.8mg.

Ingredients:

- ¼ cup of plain yogurt

- 1½ teaspoon of brown sugar

- 1 pear, diced

- 1 apple, diced

- 1 cup of sliced celery (Optional)

- ½ cup of raisins

- ¼ cup of dried cranberries

- 2 tablespoons of chopped walnuts

- 1 dash of ground cinnamon (optional)

- 1 dash of ground nutmeg (optional)

Instructions:

1. To make a dressing, blend the yogurt and brown sugar in a bowl.

2. In a cup, blend the peach, apple, cranberries, celery, raisins, and walnuts.

3. To mix, add dressing and toss properly. Sprinkle the end with cinnamon and nutmeg.

4. Before serving, cool the salad for at least 30 minute.

Chapter 9: Dessert Recipes

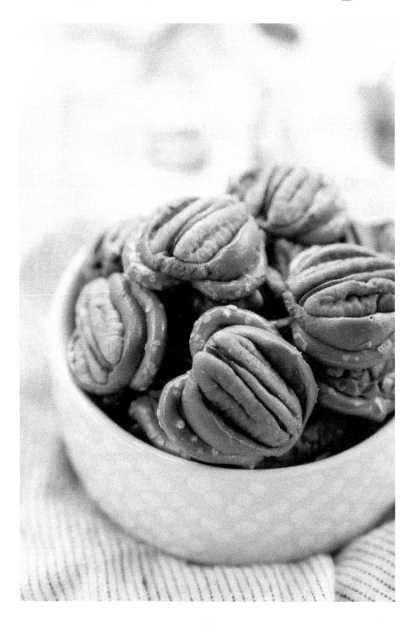

In this chapter, we are going to give you some delicious and mouthwatering recipes

On Lean & Green Dessert recipes.

47. Pretzel Turtles®

(Ready in 14 Minutes, Serve 20, Difficulty: Easy)

Nutrition per Serving:

Calories 182, Protein 1.7 g, Carbohydrates 14.1 g, Fat 2.2 g, Cholesterol 0.4mg, Sodium 262.9mg.

Ingredients:

- 20 small mini pretzels

- 20 chocolate-covered caramel candies

- 20 pecan halves

Instructions:

1. Preheat the oven to 300 degrees Fahrenheit (150 degrees Celsius).

2. Arrange the pretzels on a parchment-lined baking sheet in one single layer. On each pretzel, put one chocolate-covered caramel candy.

3. For 4 minutes, bake. Press ½ pecan onto each candy covered pretzel when the candy is soft. Cool absolutely in an airtight jar before storage.

48. Sarah's Applesauce

(Ready in 30 Minutes, Serve 4, Difficulty: Easy)

Nutrition per Serving:

Calories 121, Protein 0.4 g, Carbohydrates 31.8 g 1, Fat 0.2 g, Cholesterol 0mg, Sodium 2.7mg.

Ingredients:

- 4 apples, peeled, cored, and chopped

- ¾ cup of water

- ¼ cup of white sugar

- ½ teaspoon of ground cinnamon

Instructions:

1. Combine the apples, water, sugar, and cinnamon in a saucepan.

2. Cover and simmer for 15-20 minutes over medium heat, or until the apples are tender. Allow it to cool, then mash it with a potato masher or fork.

49. Fruity Fun Skewers

(Ready in 15 Minutes, Serve 5, Difficulty: Easy)

Nutrition per Serving:

Calories 61, Protein 0.9 g, Carbohydrates 15.4 g, Fat 0.3 g, Cholesterol 0mg, Sodium 5.1mg.

Ingredients:

- 5 large strawberries, halved

- ¼ cantaloupe, cut into balls or cubes

- 2 bananas, peeled and cut into chunks

- 1 apple, cut into chunks

- 20 skewers

Instructions:

1. Thread the bits of strawberries, cantaloupe, banana, and apple alternately onto skewers, putting on each skewer at least 2 pieces of fruit. On a serving platter, place the fruit skewers decoratively.

50. Barbequed Pineapple

(Ready in 8 Hours and 30 Minutes, Serve 4, and Difficulty: Easy)

Nutrition per Serving:

Calories 151, Protein 0.8 g, Carbohydrates 30.9 g 1, Fat 0.4 g, Cholesterol 0mg, Sodium 6.1mg.

Ingredients:

- 1 fresh pineapple

- ¼ cup of rum

- ¼ cup of brown sugar

- 1 tablespoon of ground cinnamon

- ½ teaspoon of ground ginger

- ½ teaspoon of ground nutmeg

- ½ teaspoon of ground cloves

Instructions:

1. Peel the pineapple and cut off the middle core, thus leaving it whole. Slice them into 8 rings and place them in a resealable plastic bag or shallow glass dish. Mix the bourbon, brown sugar, cinnamon, ginger, nutmeg, and cloves in a shallow dish. 2. Pour over the pineapple marinade, cover it, and refrigerate for 1 hour or overnight.

Preheat the high-heat barbecue. Slightly grated gasoline.

3. Pineapple rings are grilled for 15 minutes, rotating once or until dried, and char marked around. Serve with the marinade that remains.

Conclusion

The Lean & Green diet can undoubtedly help you lose weight as well as keep it off because its meals are lower in fat and cholesterol, and the foods called "fuelings" contain a good amount of high-quality soy or whey protein to meet your daily nutritional requirements. The help of coaches is essential while you are on the diet, as you will have the opportunity to be part of a support group. Once the target weight is reached, the new healthy habits will replace the old ones and you will be able to maintain your weight and good health.

The "Lean & Green" diet combines meals and a nutritious snack, such as a serving of fruit or a small snack, for those who are looking for a more versatile or higher calorie diet or simply to maintain their ideal weight. For best results, it is recommended to perform low-intensity physical activity for at least 30 minutes, including walking or swimming, or whatever you like, as long as it is done without exaggerated efforts. Besides, you should avoid all refined cereals, sugary drinks, fried foods, and alcohol. It is about having a low carbohydrate intake through pre-packaged meals and lean proteins and non-starchy vegetables.

Lightning Source UK Ltd.
Milton Keynes UK
UKHW022002020421
381458UK00003B/111